Title: Aari's Fruit-Tastic Colors
Author: Aariyah Cobb
Illustrator: GiGi

Copyright: © 2024 Oluchi Coaching and Consulting, LLC
All Rights Reserved.

ISBN Print: 979-8-9866001-5-4

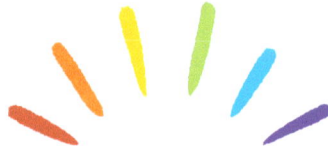

Aariyah's Biography

Aariyah Cobb, a remarkable seven-year-old, is already making waves with her debut children's book aimed at promoting healthy eating habits among her peers. As a third grader on the honor roll, Aariyah's intelligence shines brightly in everything she does. She is not only smart, creative, and witty but she also radiates beauty and talent of drawing and designing clothes for her dolls out of balloons. Her love for learning is evident in her daily activities, and she approaches each day with a spirit of curiosity and enthusiasm.

With aspirations of becoming a doctor one day, Aariyah hopes to continue her journey of helping others maintain good health. She desires to make a positive impact on the world. Aariyah a.k.a "Aari the Legend" is a name to remember, as she continues to inspire and uplift those around her with her kindness, intelligence, and unwavering determination.

Dedication

This book is dedicated to my GiGi who helped me to make my dream come true of being a children's author. She always keeps her promises with me. She is the best GiGi in the world, and I love you sooo sooo much! Thank you GiGi!

I would also like to make a dedication to my wonderful mommy who brought me into his world, and shaped me into the amazing young girl that I am. I promise that I will make you proud one day. I love you sooo soo much!

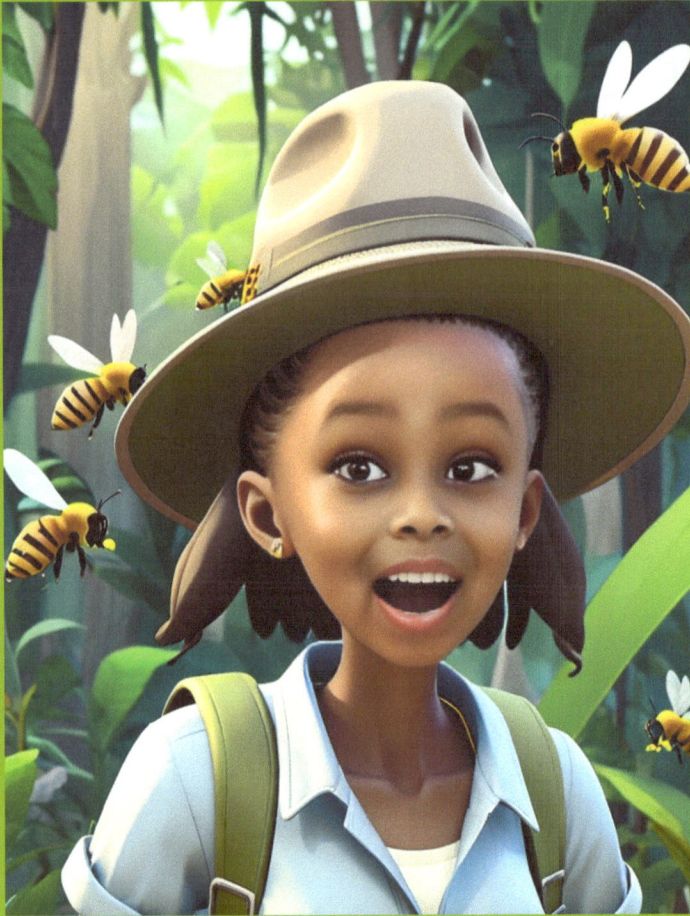

Hi! Im Aari,

Welcome to the wonderful world of colorful fruits.

Are you ready to go on a Fruit-tastic journey with me?

Let's Go on a Fruity Adventure and learn about the colors of different fruits.

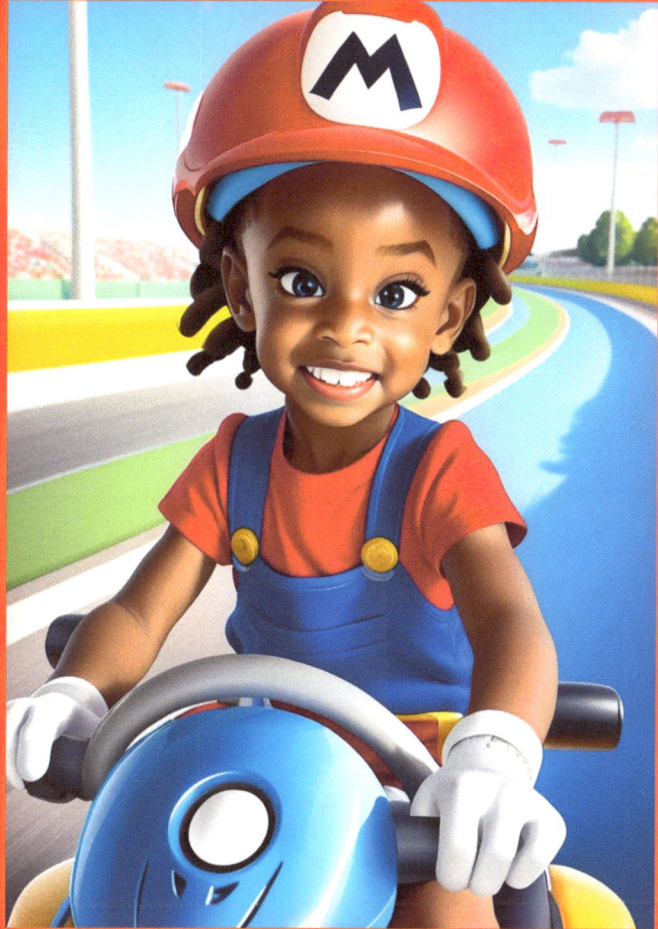

Eating Organic fruits is Super healthy and Fun! Let's Start with the color Red.

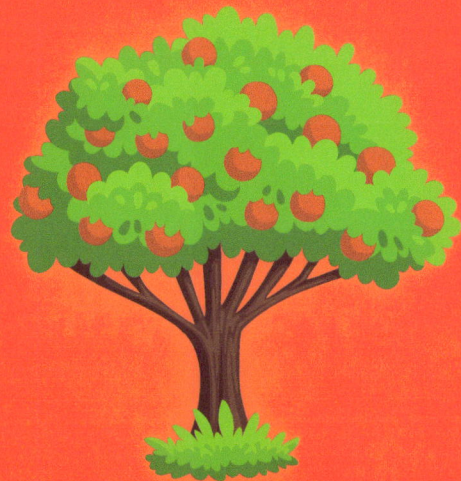

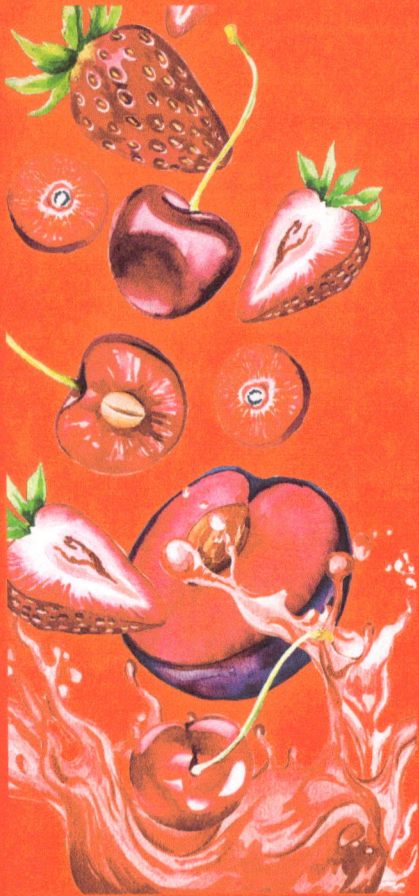

What does the "red" color in fruits mean?

Red fruits are colored by a chemical compound called carotenoid that helps the body to resist bacteria and viral infections.

Red Fruits are good for your digestive system, the heart and your eyes.

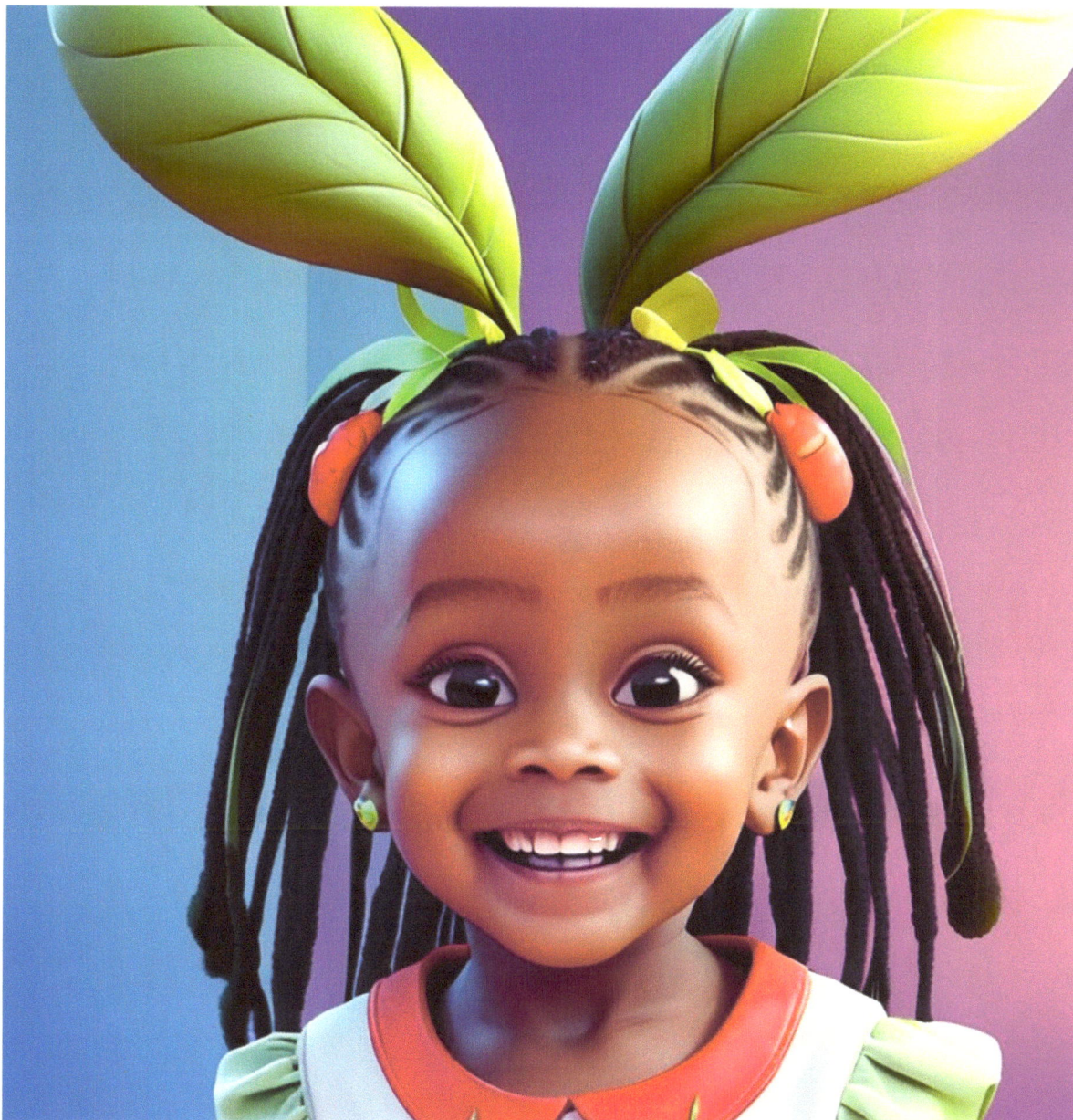

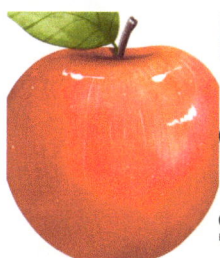

Red Apples are sweet and crunchy. They keep you strong and healthy. Yum! Can you find something else that is red?

Watermelon is **Red** on the inside. When eaten, it helps the heart to function better. The seeds in the watermelon contains fatty acids that can help to reduce cholesterol levels and regulate blood pressure levels.

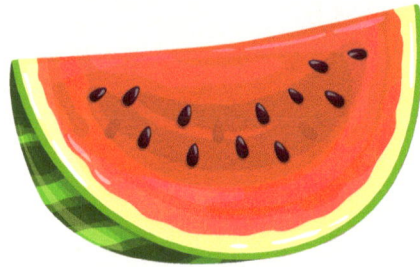

Watermelon with seeds can also help to moisturize the skin, strengthens the hair and improve the digestive system.

*Remember to tell mommy and daddy to buy the watermelon "with" seeds.

Look at this juicy Strawberry! It's also red, and it tastes Amazing!

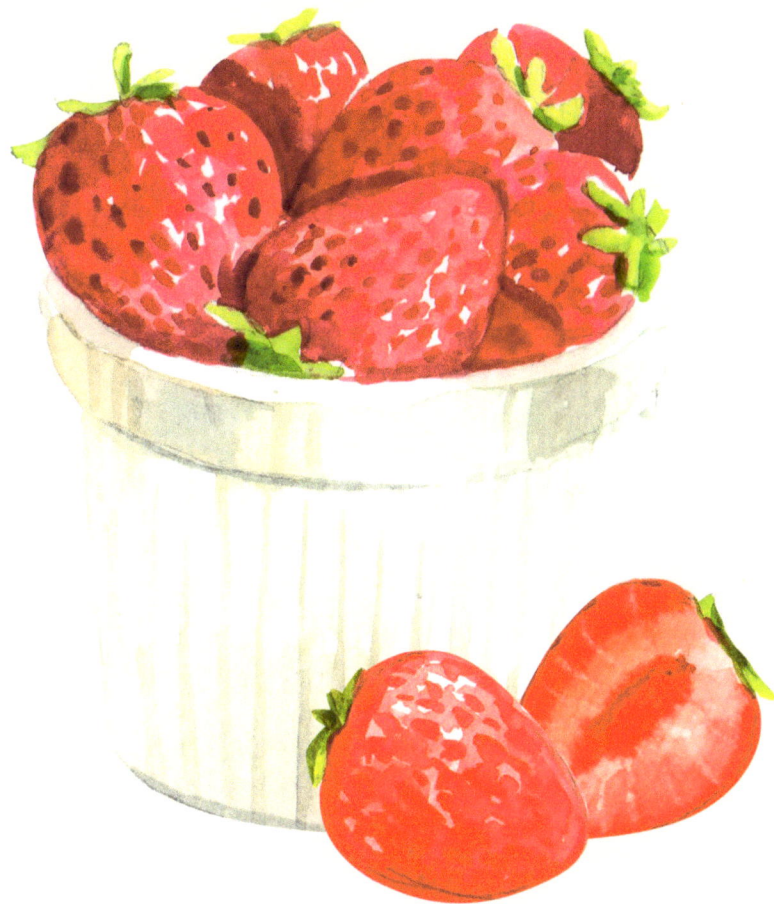

Strawberries help you to stay fit and full of energy!

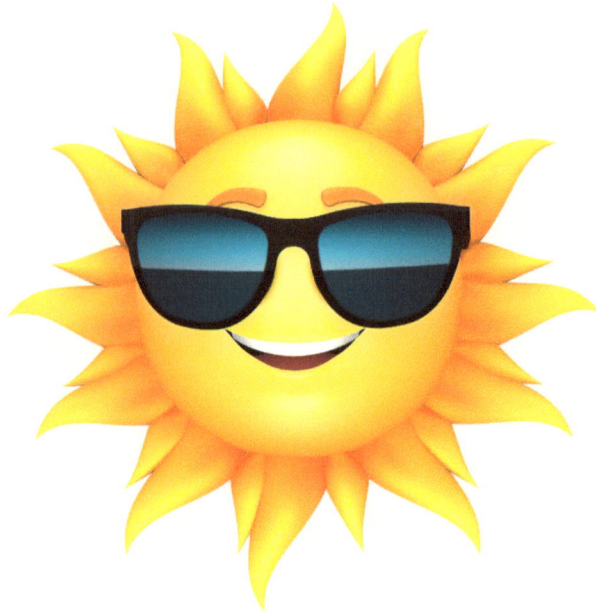

What does the "yellow" color in fruits mean?

The "Yellow" color in fruits indicates that they are ripe and nutritional.

Yellow fruit is important for vision, growth and development, skin, and immune functioning

NOW LET'S TAKE A LOOK AT SOME YELLOW FRUITS.

CAN YOU THINK OF A YELLOW FRUIT?

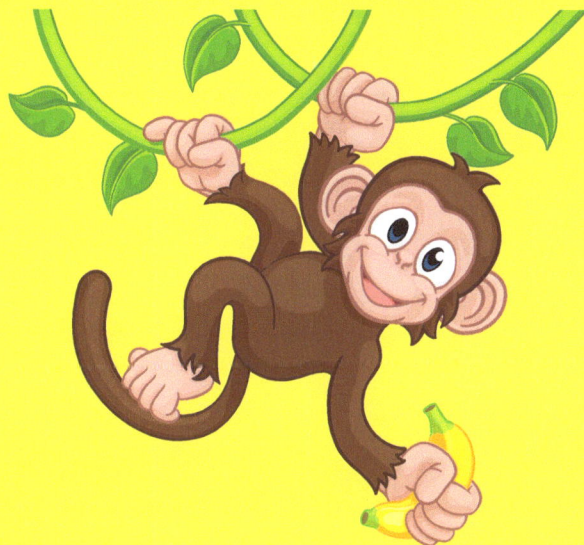

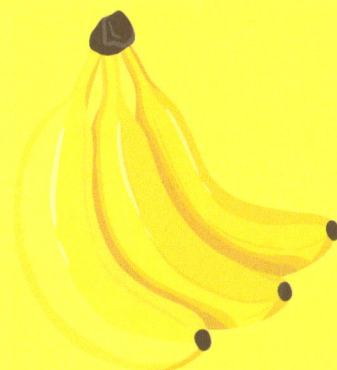

Bananas are yellow and super yummy. They give you lots of energy to play all day long. They are also good for the heart. What other yellow fruits can we find?

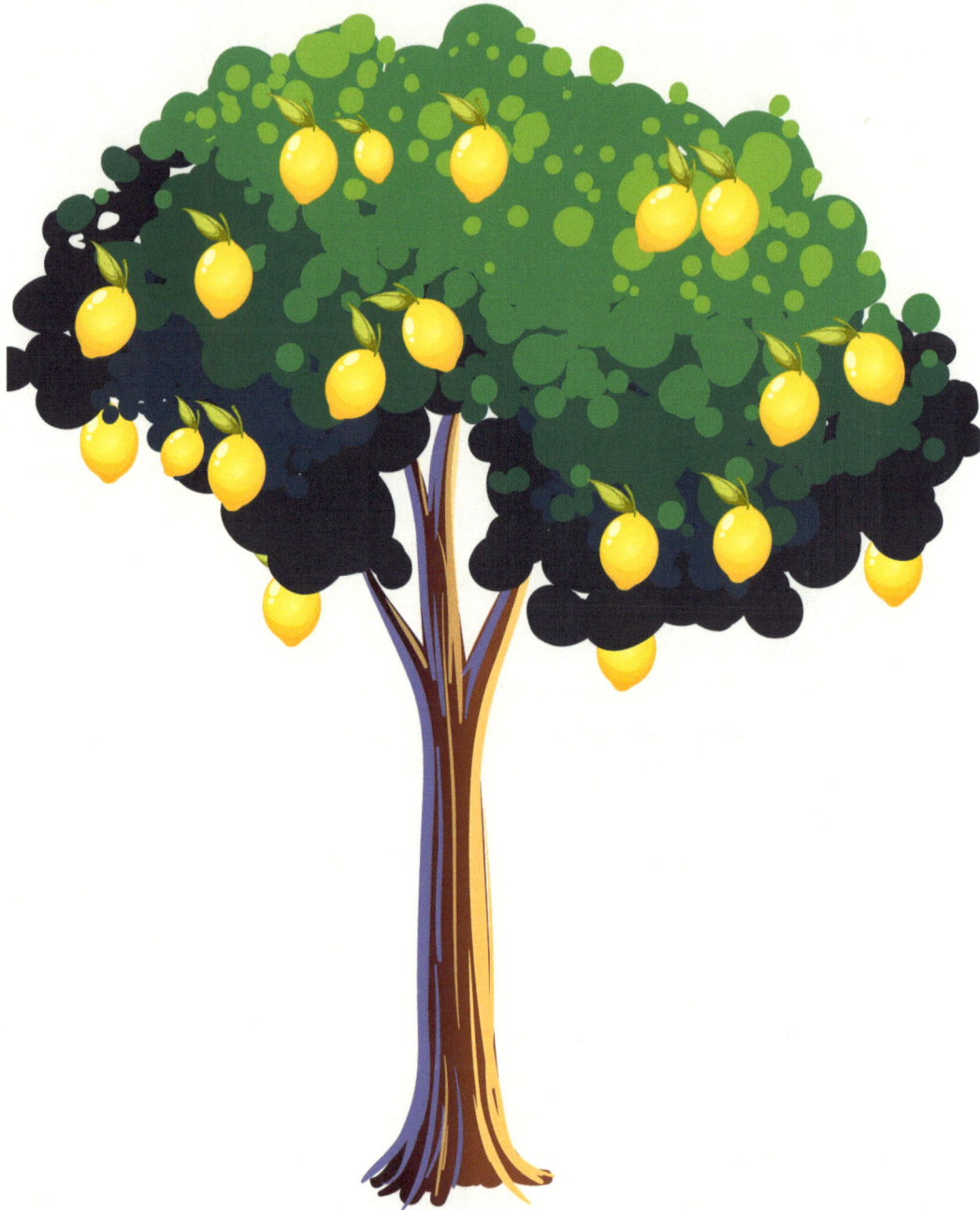

Lemons are another yellow fruit that
helps to build your immune system.
It is packed with Vitamin C.

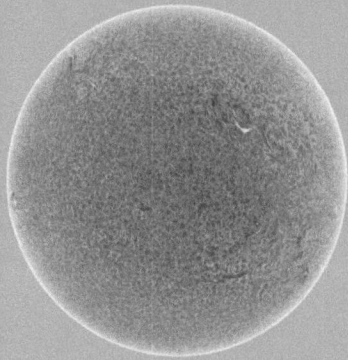

What does the "Orange" color in fruits mean?

The "Orange" color in fruits is a symbol of fertility and luxury.

On the spiritual side of the orange fruit, it represents optimism, happiness and youthful connections.

Oranges are bright and juicy. They are filled with Vitamin C, which helps you stay healthy and fight off colds.

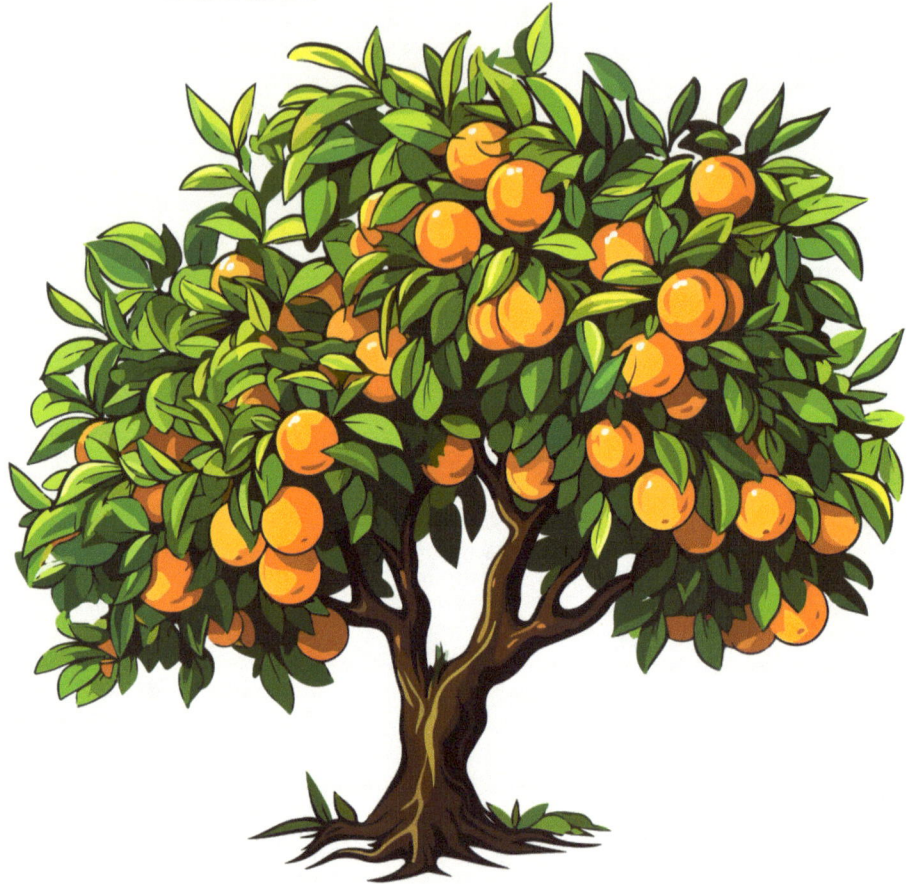

Oranges are also good for your tummy aches and other digestive issues.

What other fruit is orange?

**Peaches are orange and are
an excellent source of
Vitamin C and Fiber.**

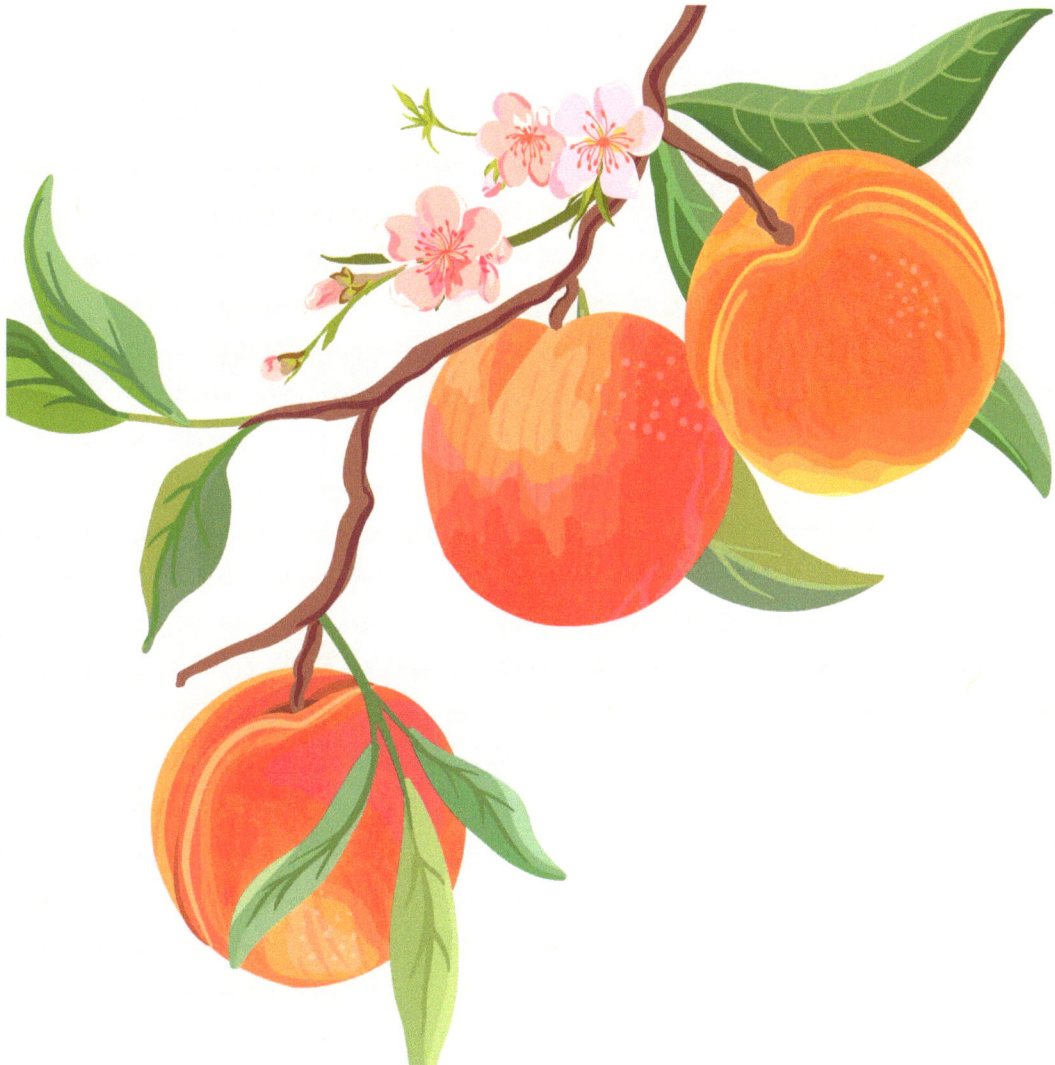

It's all Peachy!

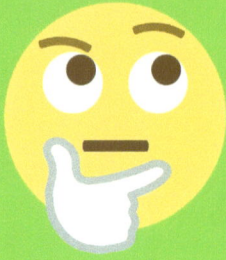

Can you guess what the "Green" color of fruits mean?

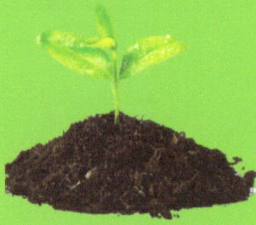

Green Fruits such as green apples, Pears, and green grapes. It contains chlorophyll which is a green pigment that plants use to make food during the photosynthesis stage.

Chlorophyll can help boost red blood cells, which can help heal damaged skin and eliminate toxins out of the body. It can also prevent cancer cells from forming and growing.

The "green" color of fruits symbolizes "wealth".

Pears are **Green** in color. They are a good source of fiber and are high in vitamins **A**, **C** and **K**. They promote gut health, and heart health.

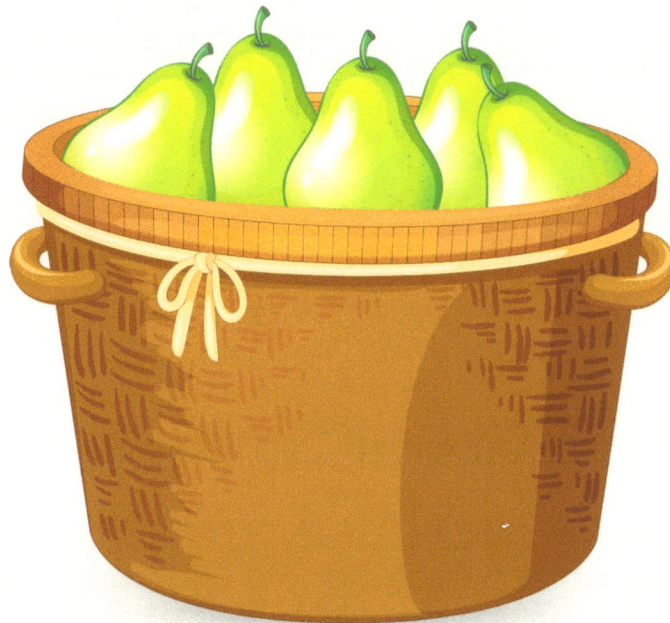

Pears can also fight against certain diseases such as heart disease, Type 2 diabetes, asthma and cancer. It also helps the body to heal faster from wounds.

Apples can also be "Green". Green apples are a good source of Vitamin C. They are high in fiber and water. They support the digestive system, the heart, the skin and the hair.

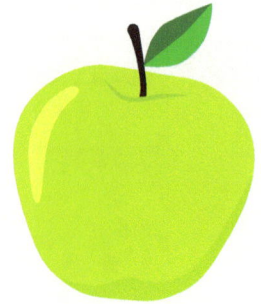

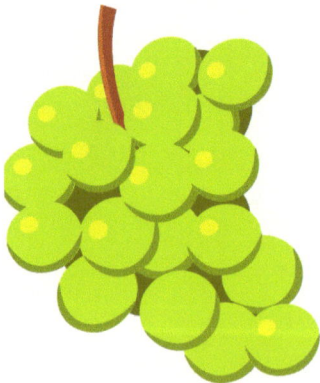

"Green" grapes helps to increase energy levels, improve heart health, eye health and bone health.

Green grapes is also a natural melatonin that can help you to sleep better.

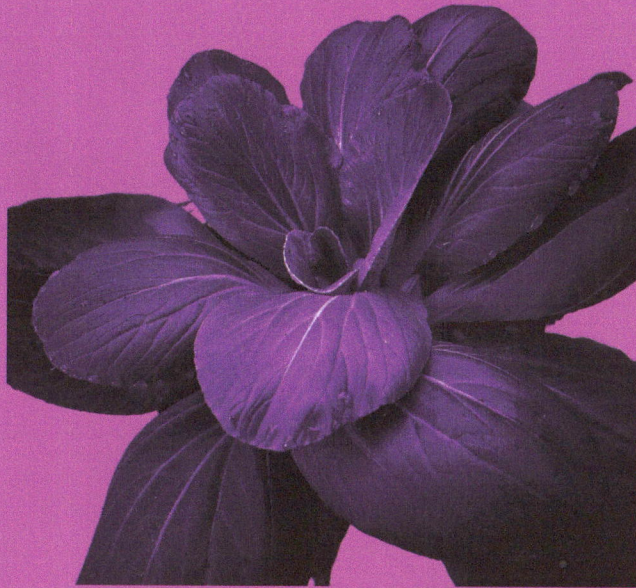

What does the "purple" color in fruits mean?

The purple color of these fruits mean that they are rich in antioxidants, which can greatly improve and prevent certain health conditions such as high blood pressure, high cholesterol, and heart and brain conditions.

16

Grapes can be "Purple".
They are good for the
immune system because
they are rich in
antioxidants, and contain
Vitamin C and K.

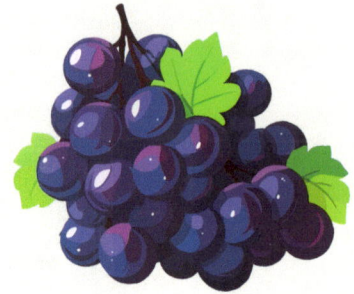

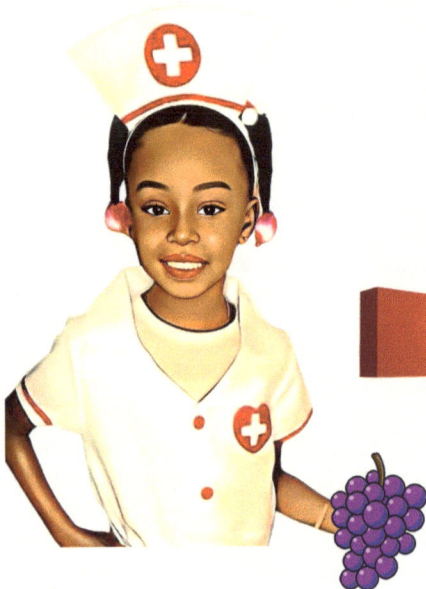

Purple grapes also
helps to improve
eye and bone
health. And...It
helps to protect
against cancer.

The seeds in purple grapes helps to
reduce inflammation in the body, and
prevent liver damage.

Plums are "Purple".
They are rich in
vitamins C and K,
antioxidants, and
minerals.

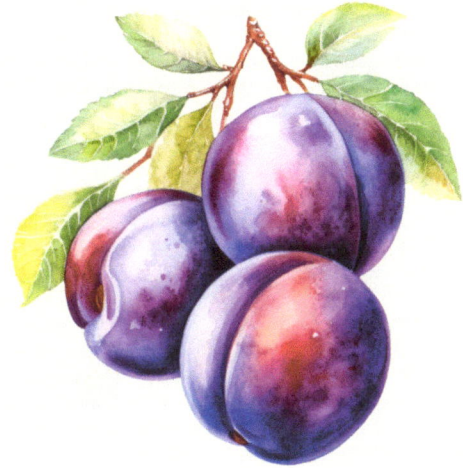

Plums help with the digestive system,
improve the brain, helps to keep your
skin healthy and can protect you
against the cold and flu.

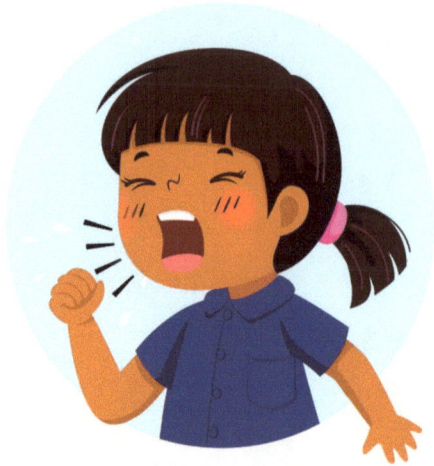

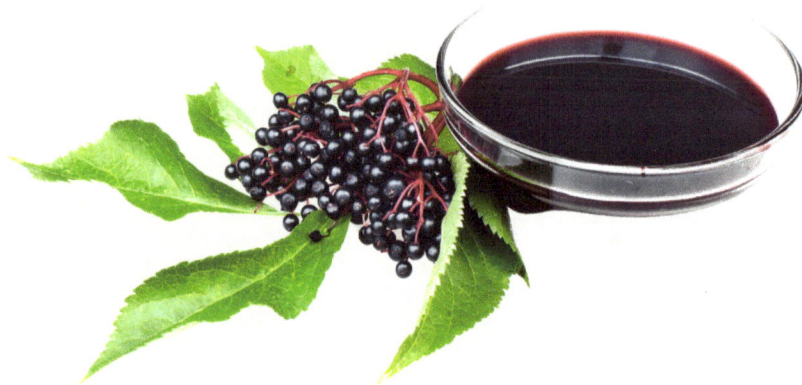

Elderberry is a "Purple" fruit that is filled with Vitamin C. It helps to fight against the common cold, flu, and inflammation in the body.

What does the "Blue" color in fruits mean?

The blue color in fruits comes from an antioxidant pigment that plants use to protect themselves from UV light and insects.

It helps to maintain urinary tract health, improve heart health and memory.

Blue fruits can also lower the risk of chronic diseases such as kidney disease, arthritis and depression.

Blueberries are "Blue".
They contain
antioxidants that help
to strengthen the
bones, improve the
immune system, and
fight against asthma
and cancer.

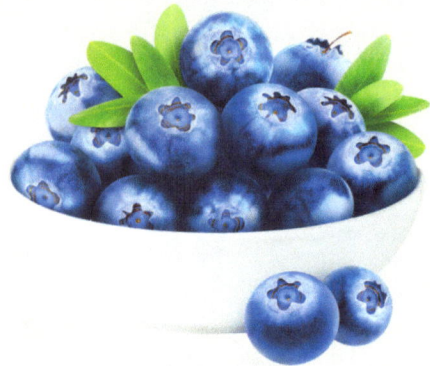

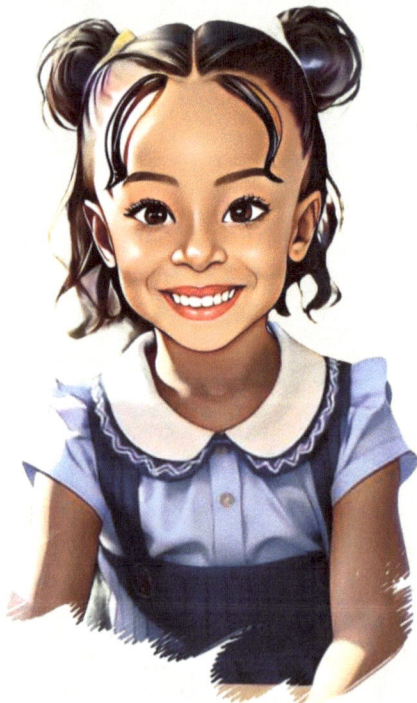

Would you like to
have a Blueberry
muffin with me?

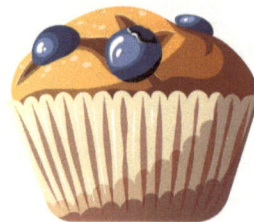

Can you tell
me what
you learned
about Fruits
today?

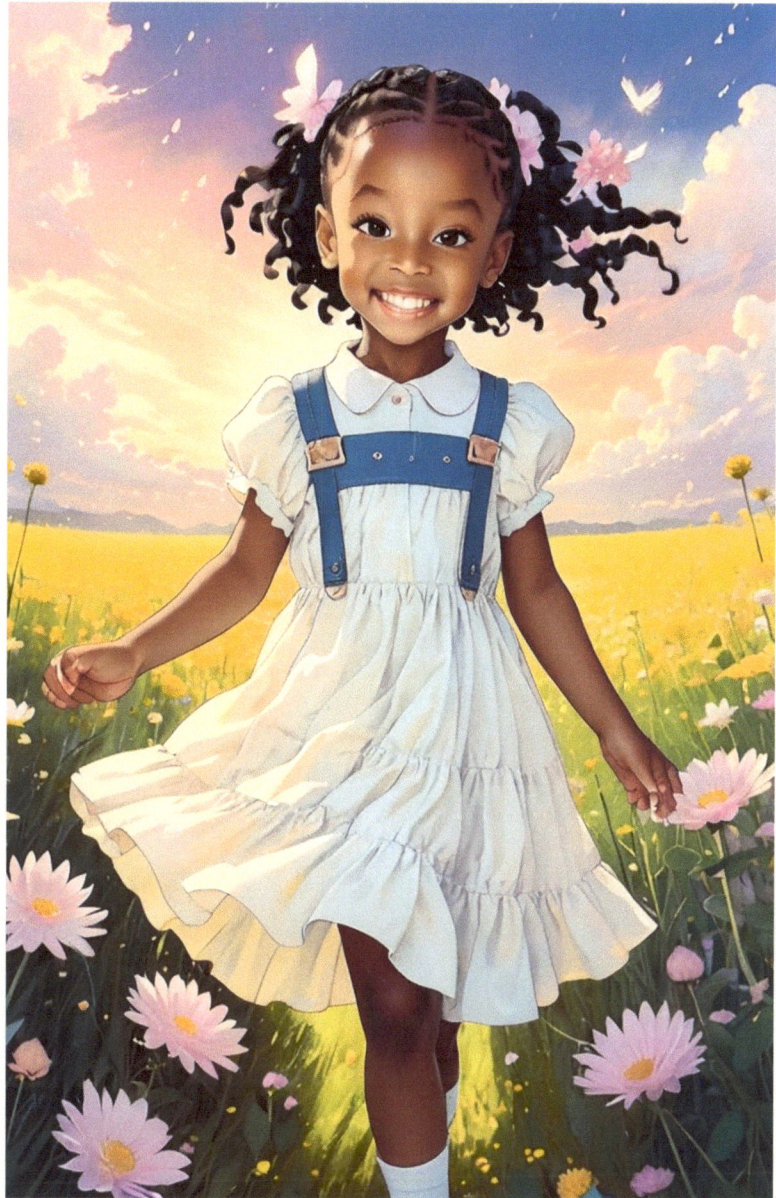

Let's Recap together.

Thank you for going on this Fruit-Tastic journey with me. We learned about the different colors of Fruit starting with the color "Red".

What types of Fruits are Red?

Apples
Watermelon
Strawberries

Yay! I'm so proud of You!

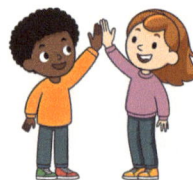

Next, we learned about the color "Yellow".

What type of fruits are yellow?

Bananas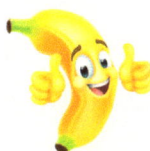

Lemons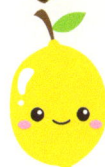

Yay! You're Amazing!

We also learned about the color
"Orange"

What types of fruits are orange in color?

Oranges

Peaches

HOORAY!

Next, we learned about the color "Green"

What types of fruits are green in color?

Pears

Grapes

Apples

Wow! You're so smart! 😍

We learned about the color "Purple"

What color fruits are purple in color?

Grapes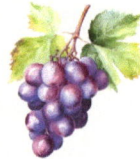

Plums

Elderberries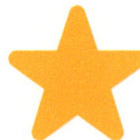

Great job! ⭐

Lastly, We learned about the color "Blue"

What color fruit are blue in color?

Blueberries

Fantastic!

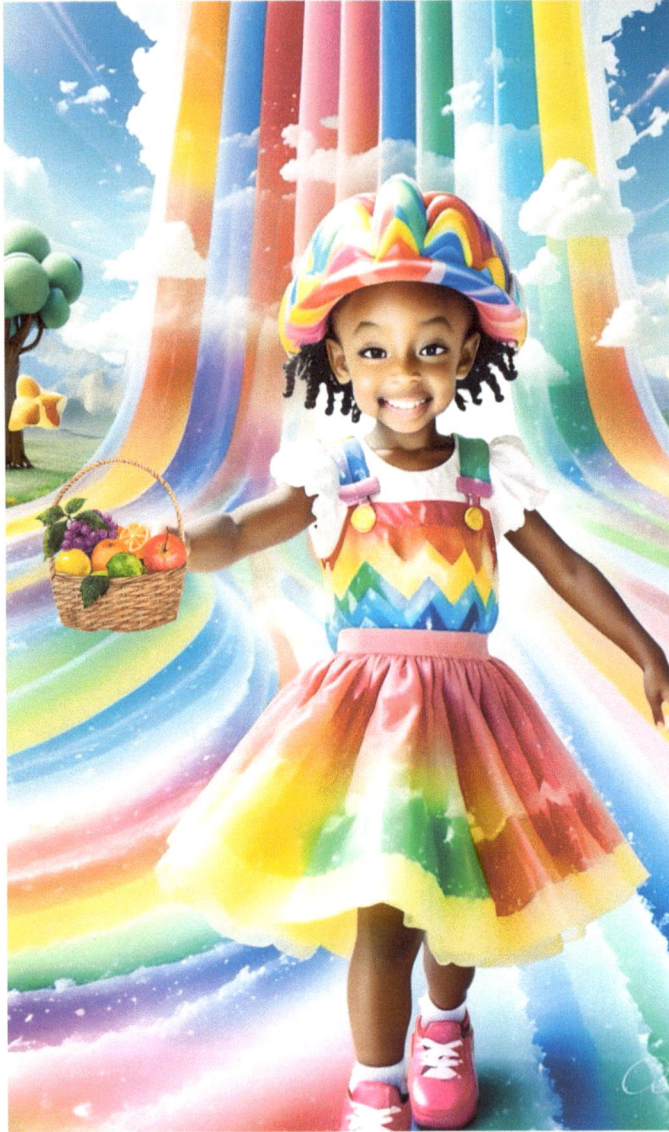

Eating a rainbow of fruits keeps us healthy and strong. Organic fruits are the best because they are grown without harmful chemicals.

Remember to eat fruits every day! They make you feel great and give you lots of energy to learn and play.

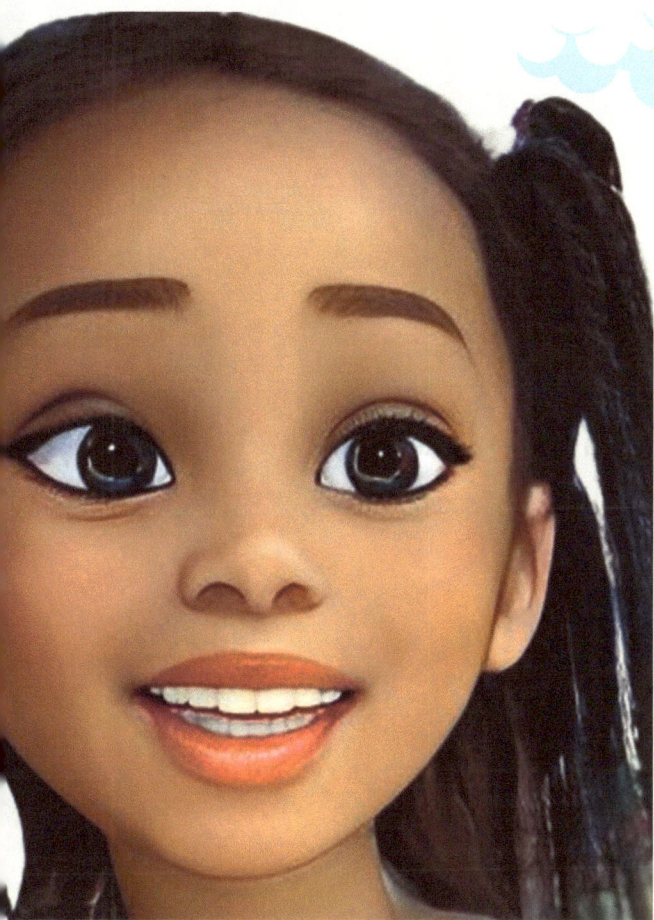

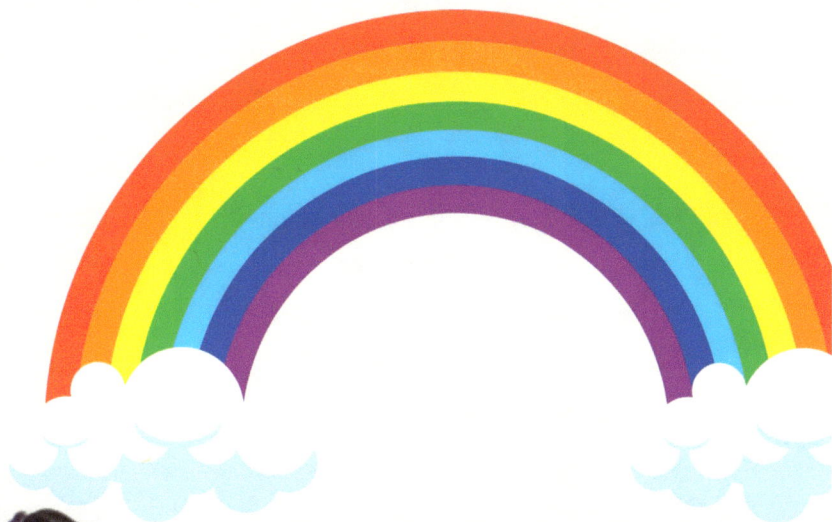

Wasn't learning fun?
I think you deserve a
fun treat.
Let's have some fun
coloring of some of
the fruit that we
learned about.

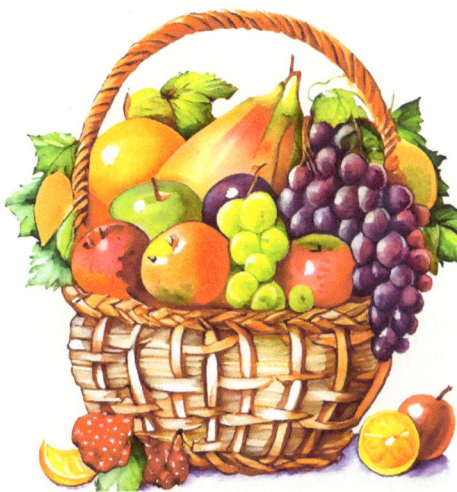

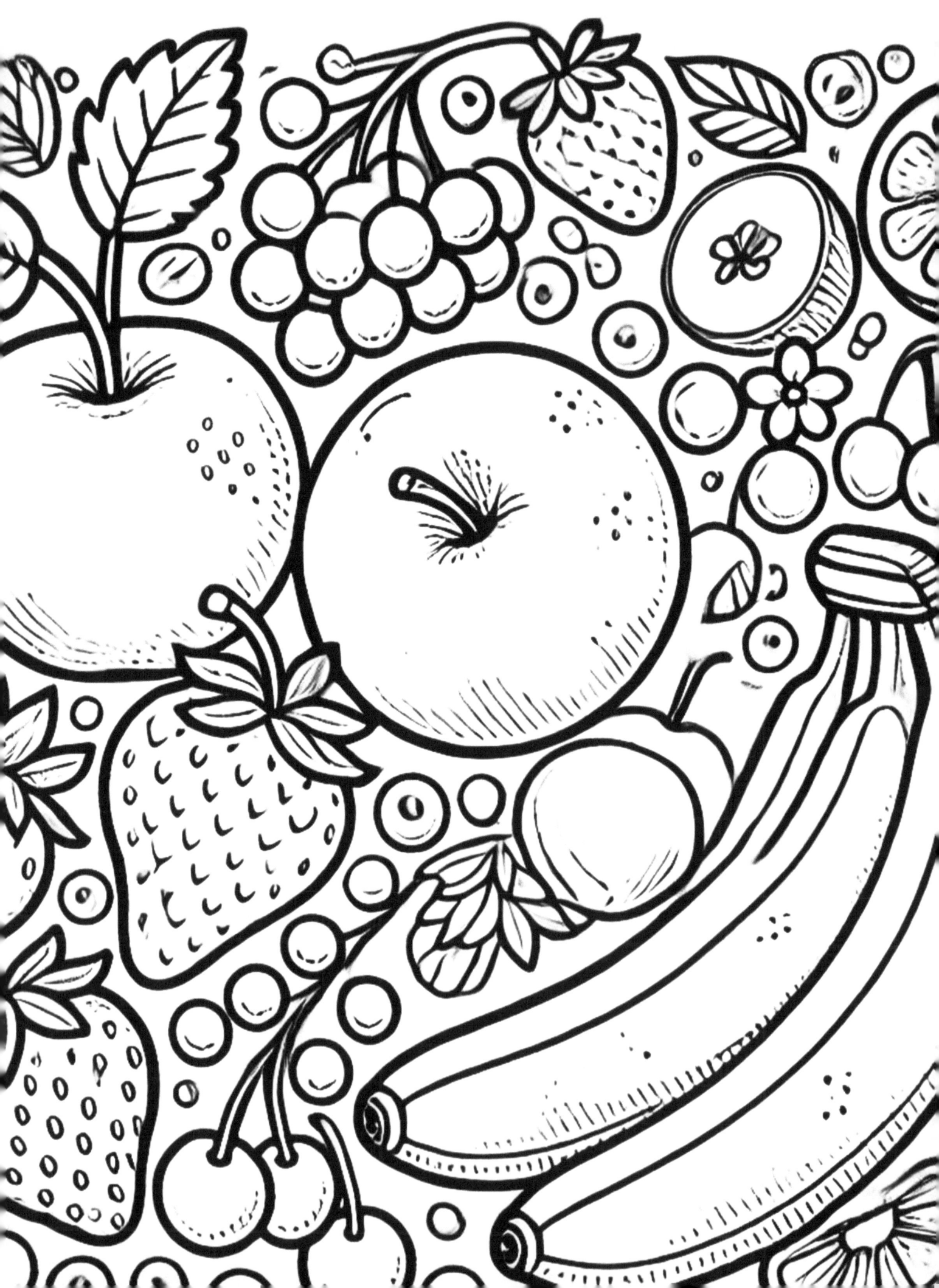

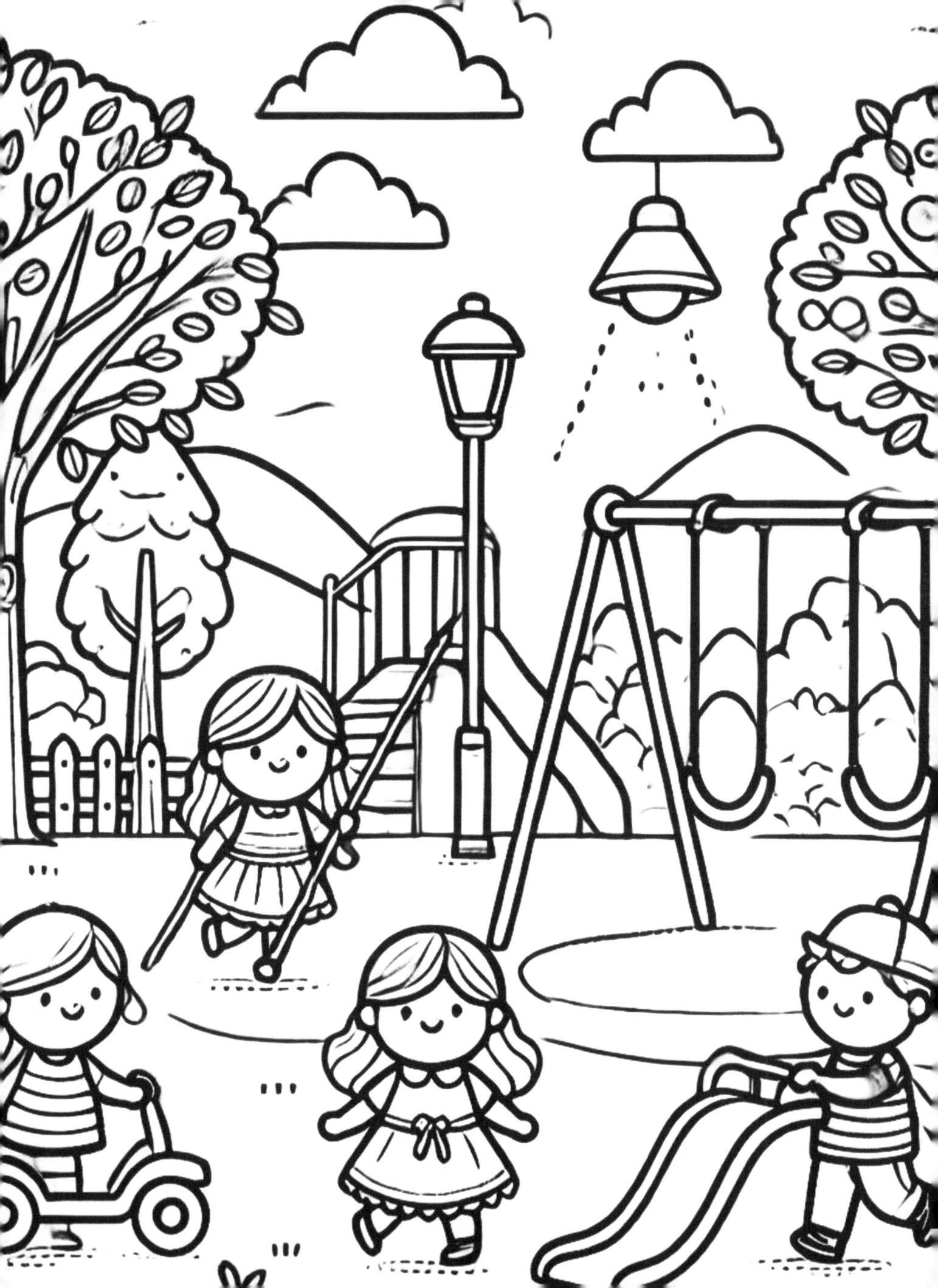

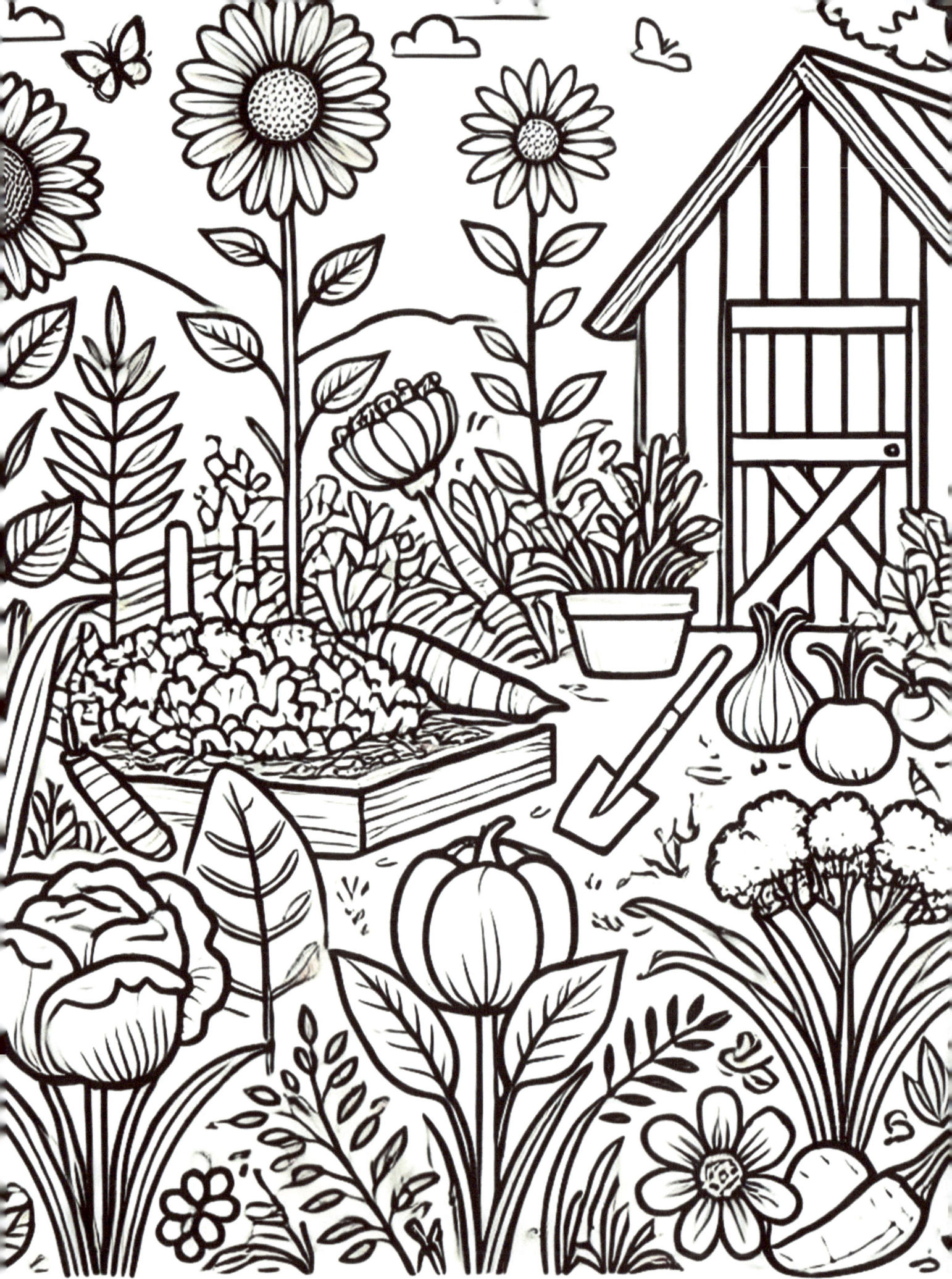

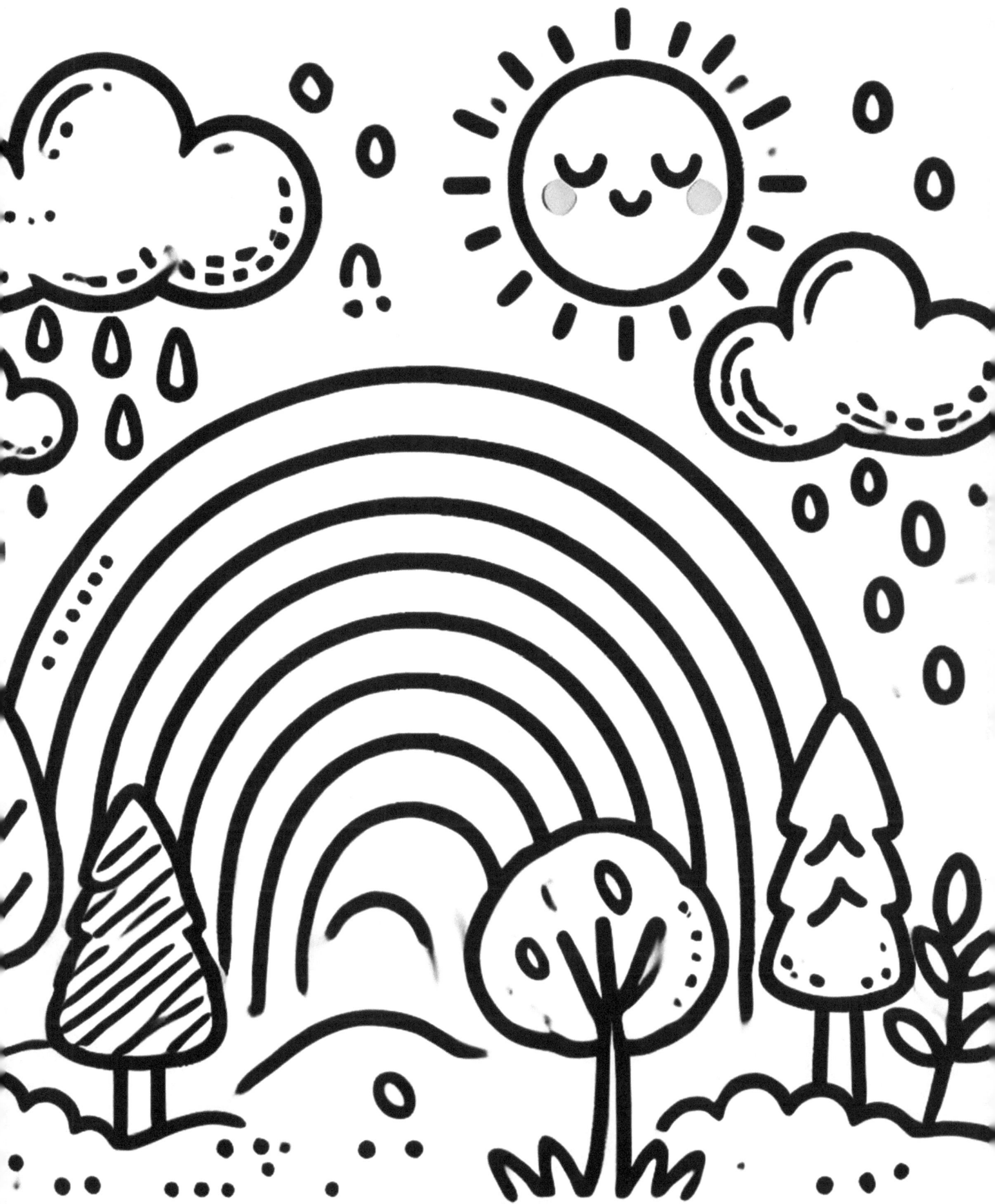

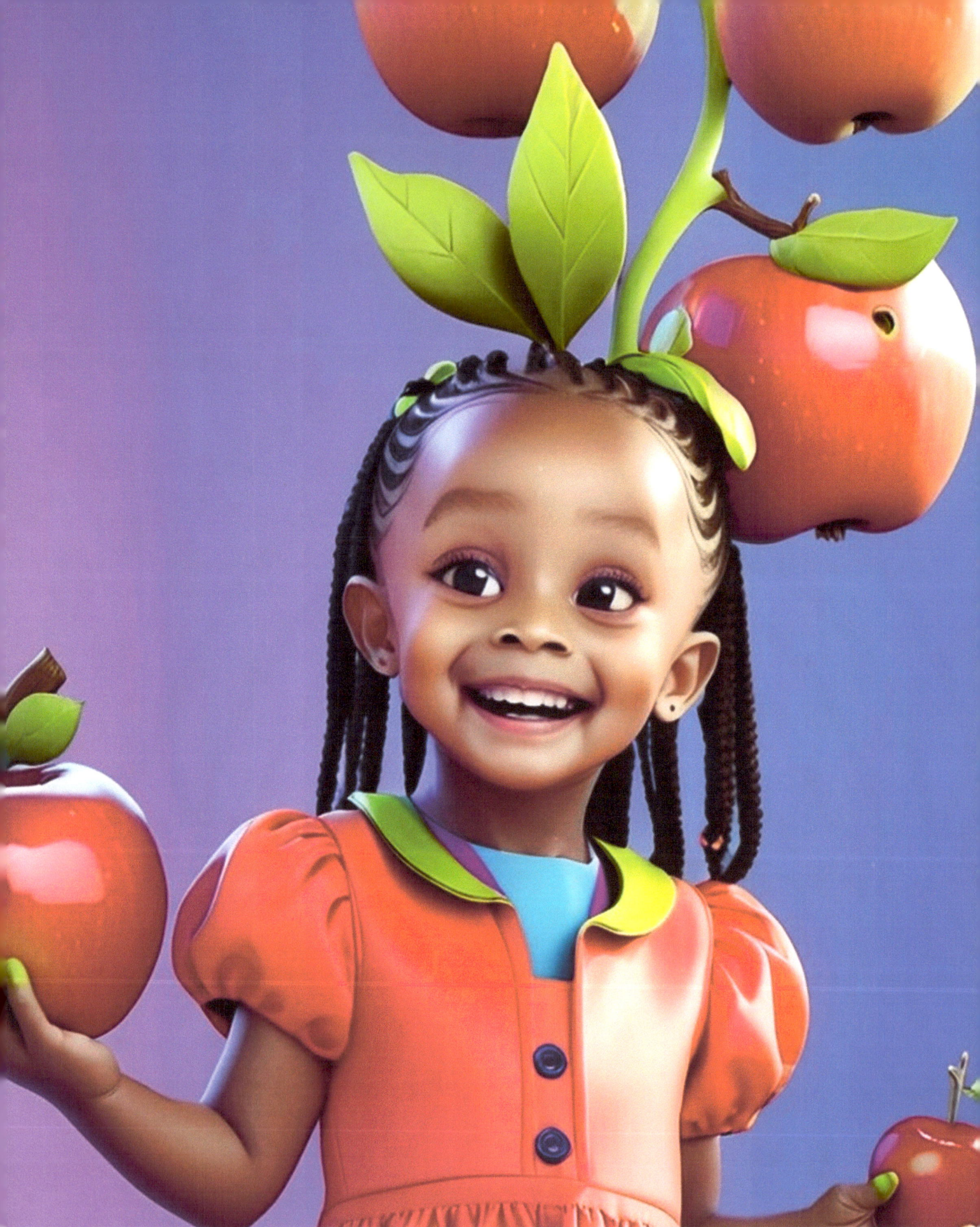

Have a Fruit-Tastic Day!

www.ingramcontent.com/pod-product-compliance
Lightning Source LLC
Chambersburg PA
CBHW061144030426
42335CB00002B/91